Strength Training For Women:

Strength, Fat and Weight Loss Workouts, Routines, Exercises and Dieting Guide

By

Charles Maldonado

Table of Contents

Introduction 5

Chapter 1. Start with The Heart 6

Chapter 2. Garbage-in Garbage-out 12

Chapter 3. The Weighting is The Hardest Part 20

Chapter 4. Workout Routine Plan 23

Conclusion 28

Thank You Page 29

Strength Training For Women: Strength, Fat and Weight Loss Workouts, Routines, Exercises and Dieting Guide

By Charles Maldonado

© Copyright 2015 Charles Maldonado

Reproduction or translation of any part of this work beyond that permitted by section 107 or 108 of the 1976 United States Copyright Act without permission of the copyright owner is unlawful. Requests for permission or further information should be addressed to the author.

This publication is designed to provide accurate and authoritative information in regard to the subject matter covered. This work is sold with the understanding that the publisher is not engaged in rendering legal, accounting, or other professional services. If legal advice or other expert assistance is required, the services of a competent professional person should be sought.

First Published, 2015

Printed in the United States of America

Introduction

Training, in general, is a more specific endeavor than most people think it is. It involves dedication, information, application, execution, as well as awareness, nutrition, and motivation. Here we will discuss some of the general concepts you'll need to be familiar with if you want to build a stronger, healthier, more functional and capable you. Take these concepts as guidelines, but don't stop there. Just like exercise is a lifelong pursuit (if you want it to be truly effective) learning as well is something we're never quite finished with. Consider this a springboard to a new, fitter, you.

Chapter 1. Start with The Heart

Your cardiovascular system is the means by which your body disseminates nutrients and eliminates waste. Without a healthy cardiovascular system, there is no hope of you developing greater strength, or burning fat, or increasing flexibility, or even of improving your posture. A good cardio program is essential to any strength training program, but can operate in conjunction with other activities to provide both a good cardio workout in addition to a strength training regime.

-Toys-

Jump ropes, hula-hoops, rollerblades, a pogo-stick...toys are a great way to boost your cardio without thinking too much about it. They let you set easily definable goals and allow you to 'beat your record' the next time around. Plus, they really work. Jumping rope remains one of the most effective cardio exercises you can do, and all for the price of a piece of clothesline. The point is, mix up your cardio workout by splicing in some more fun, less structured activities, and it will become easier to work out a little every day.

-Workout a little every day-

If you're serious about improving your condition, you need to incorporate your training into your everyday lifestyle. Go for a jog every night, or jump a little rope, follow along with an aerobics routine. You'll of course create days in your exercise plan that have *real* workouts, but a little bit of cardio should find itself seeping into your everyday activities. Get a dog and go play each day…or play with the dog you have, or a neighbors. These types of exercises should be easy and fun and comprise only 30 minutes to an hour of your time. The point is that it's all about developing a healthier lifestyle. Paddleboarding, jogging, even a brisk walk at lunch time can all elevate your heart rate.

-About Heart Rate-

Now, you don't need to get overly involved in making calculations, but you should be aware of the benefits and risks of elevating your heart rate. To begin with, you need to calculate your maximum heart rate, which is a statistical prediction of the maximum rate, in beats per minute, that you should elevate your heart to without incurring much risk of detrimental effects.

To calculate YOUR maximum heart rate (MHR) begin with your age. Multiply your age by the number 0.685

That is: (age) X (0.685) = number A

Next   use   205.8 – (number calculated from above A)

So that is: 205.8 – (ageX0.685) = MHR in beats per minute.

Example: Elizabeth is 39 years old.   Therefore Elizabeth calculates her MHR as

205.8 – (39 X 0.685) → 205.8 – 26.715 = 179.085 → 179 Beats Per Minute

This is a rough estimate, but hop on the treadmill and run until you get your heart-rate up around your maximum, and it will work as a guideline for the rest of your exercise routine.

A low level cardio episode should put you somewhere around 50-60% of your MHR. Now, depending on your condition, health, weight, strength, experience, etc. you will require a different level of exertion to reach that target point. Experiment a little and find out what works for you. These are the little things you should do each day just to give your heart a little boost, to keep up your mood, increase your metabolism, burn fat, feel better, and improve overall health.

A mid-level cardio experience will put you somewhere in the range of 60-70% of MHR. This is the zone where you burn fat. Exercise at this level will leave you feeling slightly winded and should generate a sweat. For someone Elizabeth's age, provided they are in moderately good condition, this type of exercise would be an extended jog, a spirited bike ride, a good swim, or some fairly low energy aerobics.

Next, at 70-80% MHR, you enter the aerobic zone. Extended training in the aerobic zone is the surest way to improve your endurance. To see if you are functioning in this zone, try the 'talk-test'. You should be able to say a short sentence without gasping, but you should be burning a good deal. Recovery should still come pretty rapidly (if not, it will after another week or two training at this level). Sweat will flow pretty regularly while operating in this zone, and when working at this level, both warm-up and cool-down periods become essential to avoid pulling a muscle or cramping up.

Finally, we have the anaerobic zone. This is around 80-90% of your MHR threshold and this is when you're really cookin. You will be gasping for air, your muscles will burn, and you will not be able to spend much time working in this zone. This is as far as you should push your workout. It is dangerous and unhealthy to push yourself beyond this point, and should only do so with the clearance of a medical professional and under the guidance of an experienced trainer. This is where professional athletes push themselves occasionally and really, there's no reason for you to consider it. In fact, it's unlikely that you'll be able to imagine pushing yourself beyond the aerobic zone with some professional guidance.

Overall, you should enter a low-to-mid level cardio state every day if you're serious about becoming healthier. It will increase your bodies efficiency and help you maximize the results from every other activity you perform. We'll take a look later at how to integrate a cardio program into your overall strength training program in order to maximize results.

Bear in mind, that this is a guideline. Once you start working out regularly, you'll know where you stand…I mean, you'll know at what level you are working. It certainly is not necessary to be counting your heart rate and breaking out a calculator just to get an effective workout. It is necessary, to understand that your body behaves differently at these different levels, and that all of them should be incorporated into your fitness regimen.

Chapter 2. Garbage-in Garbage-out

You need to improve cardio, because that's the way your body distributes and allocates resources as well as removing waste. In order to make use of that healthy cardiovascular system of yours, it is essential to fuel your body with healthy and useful ingredients. Let's take a look at what we put in our bodies in order to make smart decisions regarding our diet. **Remember having a healthy diet is far healthier and much more rewarding than being on a diet**

-Vitamins-

How many people do you know that take vitamin supplements? And how many people do you know that can actually tell you what a 'vitamin' is? The things we call vitamins are complex macronutrients derived from nature (or created in our own bodies). They aid our bodies in completing functions that they could not perform unassisted. This is why vitamins are important. Without the proper supply, in the proper forms, coupled with their appropriate partners, our bodies cannot perform to their peak efficiency.

Interestingly, a number of recent studies show that vitamin supplements do very little to provide our bodies with the raw ingredients we truly need. This is because many of the vitamins in supplements are chemically different than found in their natural state. They are a more stable, or post-oxidized form of the molecule. Often times, we need this oxidative action for the vitamins to perform their role within our bodies. For this reason, your best bet for providing yourself with the necessary array of vitamins to live a rich and healthy life, is to follow a varied diet.

Consume a wide variety of plant foods. Consume a variety of fruits and vegetables. It's a pretty safe rule-of-thumb to assume that if a food comes in a strange color, has a unique taste, grows in an odd formation, or comes from an exotic place, that it will contain at least one strange ingredient that your body will find a use for. This takes the guess work out of your diet…just mix it up, eat mostly plant foods, and keep variety and volume very high.

-Minerals-

Minerals are exactly what they sound like…same stuff rocks are made of. When we find minerals in plants, fungi/algae, and animal foods, they are in a more useable state (which is one reason we don't eat rocks...that and the dentist bills). There are a wide array of 'micro-nutrients' our body needs, and these are typically the more rare minerals. Zinc, arsenic, iodine, and cadmium are all minerals that are toxic at low levels, but beneficial at a micro-level. We need these potential toxic substances to be truly healthy. Relax though, as long as your diet is rich and varied, there is no risk of you overdosing on iodine from a regular healthy diet.

Here, a special note on calcium –we all know it's something for women to pay particular attention to- There are studies showing that consuming calcium in the presence of protein (think of your dairy foods- milk, cheeses, yogurt, etc) the result is synergistic and actually results in higher calorie burning in addition to a healthy source of useable calcium. But, of course not all your calcium need come from dairy sources, and if weight-loss is not a concern of yours, you can skip the dairy altogether if you like.

Some other foods high in useable calcium include, all your dark-leafy greens: kale, collards, mustard, rucola, turnip greens etc. Dried figs pack a good dose of calcium, as do most cabbages (including Bok Choy). Some fish, especially trout, salmon, perch, and sardines can provide you with a great blast of protein to go along with your bone-building calcium. Additionally, you may consider almonds, sesame seeds, seaweed, oats, soy products (especially enriched), and even oranges. Now you are beginning to see, that although calcium intake should be a priority (even at a young age) a rich and varied diet provides ample opportunity to consume as much as needed in order to stay healthy and balanced.

-Fats-

Now don't have that knee-jerk response to the f-word. Fats are a necessary part of our diet and without them we risk developing dystrophic conditions later in life (parkinsons). The point is to consume healthy fats and high-density lipoprotein (good cholesterol). Sources of these are conveniently delicious, including salmon, tuna, and other fatty fishes (watch your mercury intake for those of childbearing age) nuts, beans, legumes, avocados, and tofu. These, as you've probably noticed, are also fantastic sources of protein, which we need to build muscle and burn fat. Muscle burns fat! As long as the food you eat, coupled with your exercise routine, increase your muscle mass and those muscle get a chance to burn up calories, then really your fat intake is only a secondary concern. This is why a healthy diet is far more fun than a 'diet-diet'. The occasional piece of chocolate cake or ice-cream cone won't go straight to your thighs, it'll actually burn-up on its way there.

-Protein-

A steak may be delicious (if you're into that sort of thing) , but it's not exactly the type of protein you want to rely on to build a strong healthy body and mind. This is because beef muscle, while high in protein, also contains high levels of fats, and both variety of cholesterol. Additionally, the protein in beef is of a very complex form which makes it far more difficult for your body to digest and assimilate that nutrient. If we eat complex difficult to digest proteins, we actually derive less useful nutrition from them. There are also many studies suggesting that poorly digested complex protein, when it enters the lower digestive system, may be a leading cause of inflammatory intestinal diseases, poor nutrient absorption and malnutrition disorders, and possibly even cancers of the lower digestive tract and colon.

Better options are simpler animal proteins such as chicken, pork (believe it or not) and of course fish. If you think you don't like fish, then you haven't tried enough if it. Fish isn't 'fishy' and it can be prepared, served, and eaten in so many different ways that the statement 'i don't like fish' sounds as silly as saying 'I don't like rice'. Nonsense! A quick note on pork; it got a bad rap in the 90's, in part due to the beef lobby. Pork is a simpler protein and though we associate it with fattiness, lean cuts are actually far healthier for you than beef (in most cases) Maybe it's the 'other white meat' but another way to think of it is 'the healthier red meat'. Eggs too have gotten some bad press over the years...protein vs cholesterol vs good cholesterol etc. The fact is that eggs offer all 9 essential amino acids, a rich and highly digestible form of protein, and a wide array of micro nutrients. With eggs, moderation is key. If you have no cholesterol issues and you are mostly healthy, there is no reason not to include eggs in your varied and healthy diet. On average, one egg per day, yolk and all, will provide you with the benefits you seek, without the extra cholesterol you want to avoid.

Healthier still than the simpler animal proteins, we have proteins from the plant world. Beans, nuts, legumes (peanuts, soy, lima beans) are all wonderful sources of rich, simple, readily assimilated protein. By including these foods in your daily diet, you can ensure not only enough protein to build lean strong sleek muscle, but also include enough fiber in your diet to ensure digestive health as well. A good rule would be to eat meat as a treat, and use plants as the root of your nutrition.

WAIT!!! We forgot one...the often overlooked fungi and algae foods. These too can provide protein, though not as much as the other groups. In addition, they are chock-full of some of nature's most bizarre compounds. It's no coincidence that mushrooms factor so prominently in the holistic health diets of some many ancient and long lived civilizations. Algae is like the fungi of the sea (in diversity at least) and can also provide a healthy source of iodine, necessary for thyroid health. The fungi also provide a great source of insoluble protein which is fantastic for digestive health.

When it comes to a healthy diet, it's not all green salads and rice cakes (in fact these are two of the worst foods you can eat. One is a waste of time, the other is empty calories) Vary your diet, experiment, don't be afraid to try new things. Your body, and your tastebuds will thank you.

Chapter 3. The Weighting is The Hardest Part

Many women are afraid to utilize machines or free-weights in their workout strategy. Very often, this is due to the misconception that weights build bulky muscle and will make you look 'manish'. There is absolutely no truth to this. It isn't the fact that you use weights to develop muscle (essential to good posture, strength, and fat burning) that creates bulk, it's the manner in which you use them that determines the type of muscle you build.

Short compact movements build powerful compact muscles. This might not be a bad thing if you're working your glutes. These types of exercises will yield dense rounded muscles with a discernable peak upon contraction. If you want your shoulders to 'pop' a bit, consider some high-intensity shoulder exercises to get that sculpted effect. Likewise with calves, where you want that sleek cat-like look. Basically, anywhere you want a little extra definition (triceps, abs, deltoid, glutes, back) go a little higher on the weight, shorten up the length of motion for the exercise, and keep your reps a bit lower but perform more sets of each repetition.

If you want long lean muscle, weights can still be an important part of your exercise routine. Here, however, you'll want to use lighter weight (think 1-2 lbs. even) and use long, graceful movements. The weights will help to firm and tone your muscles, as well as create integrate strength. Integrated strength is the phenomenon where muscle groups learn to function together resulting in an overall stronger muscle-system. The same way that a person with body coordination will perform most tasks better than someone with isolated skills, a coordinated muscle-system will actually yield better non-specific strength than isolation exercises (biceps curls).

For long, lean muscle, try to integrate swimming into your exercise routine. Once per week at the end of your weight training circuit, a few good laps in the pool can help to increase flexibility, strengthen and elongate muscle groups, and aid the body in flushing toxins accumulated during the previous exercise periods.

For core strength, you can utilize pilates and yoga systems, but few things give a more effective whole body workout than kettlebells. This is fun because you can choose a very light-weight bell, and still get incredible results. This exercise actually does a good job boosting your cardio-levels as well, and therefore should become a part of anyone looking to build a serious integrated health routine. You can look on the internet for the basics of how to utilize kettlebells. Once you get the basics, however, you're free to play as you please. Creating new and more challenging movements is part of the fun. It is also a simple way to target areas needing greater attention.

Chapter 4. Workout Routine Plan

Now, there are countless websites (free websites) devoted to helping you plan an exercise program, whether it be a weekly routine, or a targeted approach to a specific goal over a month or even half a year. Want to get in shape for a triathlon? It's on the net...a mud-run...a walk-a-thon...you can find all the help you want (and more) all at your fingertips. What you'll soon realize is that they all have something in common. They all build slowly and incrementally towards the ultimate goals, they all use a varied approach in order to develop full-body system health, they all include alternation between muscle groups, they are all heavy in cardio, and they all encourage you to track your results. Therefore, consider this as merely an example of what a balanced program might look like.

-Day 1- Extremities: 20 minutes cardio warm-up followed by push-ups and stretching and flexibility exercises. Biceps/triceps routine (remember for maximum effectiveness, work opposing muscle groups on the same day) Consider curls, preacher-curls, reverse curls, triceps extensions, and possibly some light bench-press or military press. Between sets of arms, work your legs. Squats (weighted or unweighted) leg lifts, reverse leg curls, and lunges are all excellent. Between sets do calf-raises or push-ups to keep your heart-rate elevated and your blood pumping. Finish with a cooldown jog and some stretching

-Day 2- Crossfit: Begin with a light cardio warm-up followed by stretching. The goal of this day is to incorporate full body movements to build an integrated system. This exercise should focus on keeping your heart rate elevated to the aerobic zone for most of the workout. You'll tend to lose that 'weak-feeling' on these days, so be careful not to overdo it. Go for a variable run, alternating between a jog, a run, and a sprint. Try to vary your terrain as well. Not just in incline, but also in substrate (get off the track and run on grass, sand, in water, etc) As always, you can use push-ups as a way to rest from cardio without letting your heart-rate drop too much. Also, this is a great day for your kettlebell workout.

-Day 3- Core: Your distal muscle groups have gotten a good workout so far, and now it's time to really focus on your core. Warm up with some jump rope until loose and limber. Stretch out and get ready. Today you want to work your core. Plank positions, sit-ups, back raises, intercostal arm hangs, and even pull-ups, squat-thrusts, and arm circles can all fit into this day. Remember to perform both uni-directional as well as dual and multi-directional core exercises. The key is to control your movement and to control your breathing. You should feel these deep in your abs and back. Don't forget to strengthen the lower abdomen and pelvic floor to avoid injury (like a hernia). Finish with some light aerobics to stretch out those muscles and remove the blood-clots formed during strenuous exercise.

-Recovery Days- These can be interspersed as you feel necessary. Don't not repeat any of days 1-3 without first putting a recovery day in between. As always you'll want to warm up and stretch (if you're new to this then by now you're pretty sore). This is a good day to go for a long light jog. Yoga or other low impact, long movement based activity will serve to integrate the muscle groups, increase circulation and speed recovery. Maybe today you go for a swim, or a rugged hike on a local trail. A good light intensity bike ride is another way to promote circulation. These are not rest days, they are recovery days, and they are essential to promote health and prevent injury. Take them seriously as a part of your fitness regimen, and also make them fun and relaxing. Remember physical health and mental health go hand-in-hand.

You may choose to put a recovery day in between each workout day, or you may decide to just do them as needed, that choice is up to you. What is important is that you use these days regularly, and that your recovery activities are light-moderate in cardio requirements, promote long graceful movements, and access all the muscle groups evenly. In this way, you'll create the long, sleek, strong, integrated body you are naturally meant to have.

There is no book that can provide you everything you need to know regarding your own strength and fitness, but hopefully this one sets you off in the right direction. Learning how to get fit and stay fit should be a lifelong pursuit. As such, have patience if you get off to a less than inspired start. Once you make the first steps toward integrated health, it will likely become a lifelong friend to you, your body, and mind.

Be aware of your ability at every stage in your development; it's important to challenge yourself, but injuries can occur without warning. Always better to go slow when you are uncertain, and to consult doctor or trainer if you have any doubts or questions. In fact, it's always great to have a workout partner more knowledgeable than yourself. It doesn't necessarily have to be someone you see every day, just knowing you have someone in your corner can make a world of difference.

Oh yea... DRINK WATER...i know you've heard it a million times, but that's because it's a million times more important than anything else. It eliminates toxins, lowers blood pressure at times of peak exertion, promotes easier breathing, and flushes damaged tissue after intensive exercise. Life requires water...want to be healthier and have a better life? Give yourself plenty if water...and then a little more.

Conclusion

Choosing to live a healthier lifestyle, by focusing on cardio, nutrition, and strength training will make you more confident, more capable, more calm, and more comfortable in your own body. A good integrated exercise program allows your body to reach its natural potential, and it also creates opportunities for your body to create a whole pharmacopoeia of 'feel good' chemicals natural designed to reward you for your efforts, and minimize feelings of pain, tiredness, or negativity. Hopefully this introductory guide has provided you a bit of information, a good dose of motivation, and awakened your own person inspiration. It's never too soon and never too late to live a healthier life, and learn to love the life you live. Go get out there...run, sweat, grunt...lift weights get fit, get strong, push yourself...love yourself. You and your body deserve it.

Thank You Page

I want to personally thank you for reading my book. I hope you found information in this book useful and I would be very grateful if you could leave your honest review about this book. I certainly want to thank you in advance for doing this.

If you have the time, you can check my other books too.